Almond: Coconut:

Almond Flour & Coconut Flour - Gluten Free Cookbook for Paleo Diet, Celiac Diet & Wheat Free Diet

Emma Rose

Almond Flour Recipes for Optimal Health and Quick Weight Loss

Gluten Free Recipes for Celiac Disease, Gluten Sensitivities, and Paleo Free Diets

Emma Rose

Table of Contents

Introduction

I want to thank you and congratulate you for purchasing the book, *"**Almond Flour Recipes for Optimal Health and Quick Weight Loss**: Gluten Free Recipes for Celiac Disease, Gluten Sensitivities, and Paleo Free Diets"*.

This book contains proven steps and strategies on how to make dishes with almond flour.

Almond flour is gluten free and low carbohydrate alternative to commercial flour. It can be used for various dishes and pastries. You can surely incorporate it in your recipe without much hassle.

Using almond flour in your dishes can provide you with the nutrients not usually found in other types of flour. Try these recipes and enjoy healthier pastries and dishes.

Thanks again for purchasing this book, I hope you enjoy it! Please take some time to stop by and LIKE our Facebook page:

https://www.facebook.com/joypublishing

With gratitude,

Emma Rose

Emma Rose

Chapter 1: Almond Flour

Almond is native to the northern Indian subcontinent. The almond seed is more of a drupe than a nut. Like peaches, cherries and apricots, almond trees bears fruits with seeds inside which are commonly referred to as almond nut.

Almond flour is a popular substitute to wheat flour in baking and cooking. This is made from whole almonds with the skins removed. This is often preferred by health conscious individuals because it is gluten-free, high in fiber and low in carbohydrates. It is also an excellent source of protein. Almond flour is also rich in vitamins and minerals including magnesium, potassium and vitamin E.

Benefits of using almond flour:

Nutrients

Almond flour contains Vitamin E which can help prevent cell damage and heart disease. It also contains calcium which strengthens the bone and helps your circulatory system carry hormones throughout your body. Almond flour is also rich in potassium which can regulate your blood pressure.

Easy to Prepare

You can purchase almond flour in your local grocery or make it yourself. Just submerge the almonds in boiling water for a minute. Place in a strainer and remove the skin. Allow to dry then place in a coffee grinder or food processor. Process until it becomes very fine.

Complementary Foods

Serving dishes and pasties with almond flour can supplement the protein that you get from meat. It also balances your diet if it is served with fruits and vegetables. Almond flour can also compliment gluten free and low carbohydrate diets.

Reduces Heart Disease Risk

Almond contains high amounts of monounsaturated fats. This is the type of fat found in olive oil which is associated with good heart health. The antioxidants in the almond flour can also help keep the arteries healthy.

Chapter 2: Bread and Pancakes

Paleo Pumpkin Bread

Ingredients:

- 1 cup blanched almond
- ½ tsp baking soda
- 1 tsp nutmeg
- ½ cup roasted pumpkin
- ¼ tsp stevia
- ¼ tsp Celtic sea salt
- 1 tbsp ground cinnamon
- ½ tsp cloves
- 2 tbsp honey
- 3 large eggs

Procedure:

1. Combine the spices such as cinnamon, cloves, nutmeg, and cloves along with the almond flour and salt in a food processor.

2. Blend few times then add the stevia, pumpkin, eggs and honey.

3. Transfer the batter into a loaf pan.

4. Bake for 45 minutes at 350 degrees.

5. Allow to cool for an hour before slicing.

6. Serve alone or with your favorite spread.

Chocolate Zucchini Bread

Ingredients:

- 1 ¼ cups blanched almond flour

- ¼ tsp Celtic sea salt

- 2 large eggs

- ¼ cup honey

- ¾ cup grated zucchini

- ¼ cup cacao powder

- ½ tsp baking soda

- 2 tbsp coconut oil

- ¼ tsp vanilla stevia

Procedures:

1. Mix the cacao powder and almond flour in a food processor.

2. Blend in the baking soda and salt.

3. Add the eggs, honey, stevia, zucchini and coconut oil. Process few more times.

4. Transfer to a greased pan that is dusted with almond flour.

5. Bake in the oven for 40 minutes at 350 degrees.

6. Allow to cool for 2 hours before serving.

Paleo Banana Bread

Ingredients:

- 3 mashed bananas

- 1 tbsp vanilla extract

- ¼ cup palm shortening

- ½ tsp Celtic sea salt

- 3 large eggs

- 1 tbsp honey

- 2 cups blanched almond flour

- 1 tsp baking soda

Procedures:

1. Place the bananas, shortening, honey, vanilla and eggs in a food processor.

2. Blend the ingredients together until smooth.

3. Add the salt, almond flour and baking soda then process again.

4. Scoop the batter and place on the greased loaf pan.

5. Remove from the heat and place on top of the counter to cool.

6. Serve with your favorite coffee.

Irish Soda Bread

Ingredients:

- 2 ¾ cup blanched almond flour

- 1 ½ tsp baking soda

- 2 eggs

- 2 tbsp agave nectar

- Pinch of caraway seeds

- ¼ tsp Celtic sea salt

- ½ cup raisins

- 2 tbsp apple cider vinegar

Procedure:

1. Mix the baking soda, almond flour, raisins and salt in a bowl.

2. Combine the apple cider vinegar, agave nectar and eggs in a separate bowl.

3. Combine the wet and dry ingredients.

4. Place the dough in a parchment paper. Form into a large ball that is approximately 8 inches across and 1 ½ inches tall.

5. Use a knife to scrape half an inch of dough at the top. This should look like a cross.

6. Sprinkle the top with caraway seeds.

7. Place on top of the baking sheet.

8. Bake for 20 minutes at 350 degrees.

9. Turn off the oven but leave the bread inside for 10 more minutes.

10. Allow the bread to cool for 30 minutes before serving.

Sweet Potato Pancakes

Ingredients:

- 1 cup mashed sweet potatoes

- 2 eggs

- ½ tsp baking powder

- ½ tsp ground nutmeg

- 2 cups almond flour

- 4 tbsp almond milk

- ½ tsp vanilla extract

- ½ tsp ground cinnamon

Procedure:

1. Combine all of the wet ingredients together in a bowl. You can also place it in a food processor and blend it until you have a smooth consistency.

2. Combine the dry ingredients together. Use a sifter to ensure that they are evenly mixed.

3. Add the dry ingredients to the wet and stir.

4. Add coconut oil on the pan.

5. Spoon about 2 tablespoon of batter into the pan and spread it using your fork.

6. Cook for 2 minutes until bubbles appear.

7. Use a spatula and flip the pancakes.

8. Press down the pancake to ensure that the excess batter oozes out of the dough and thickening in a shape of a pancake.

9. Cook the pancake for another minute.

10. Plate it with honey and cinnamon.

Flapjacks

Ingredients:

- 2 eggs

- ½ tsp baking soda

- 1 ½ cups blanched almond flour

- ½ cup water

- ½ tsp Celtic sea salt

- ¼ cup agave nectar

- 1 tbsp vanilla extract

- Grape seed oil for sautéing

Procedure:

1. Combine eggs, vanilla, agave and water in a food processor and blend until it is smooth.

2. Add the salt, baking soda and almond flour into the mixture and blend again to incorporate the ingredients better.

3. Pour the oil in a pan and place over medium heat.

4. Pour the batter into the pan.

5. Flip the pancake when bubbles start to appear at the surface.

6. Remove from the heat and transfer to a plate.

7. Repeat the process until all of the batter is used.

Pumpkin Paleo Pancakes

Ingredients:

- ½ cup almond flour

- 1 tbsp ground flax seed

- Pinch of salt

- 1 tsp pumpkin pie spice

- ½ cup pumpkin puree

- 2 tbsp honey

- Coconut oil for frying

- 2 tbsp coconut flour

- 2 tbsp vanilla protein powder

- ½ tbsp cinnamon

- ¼ tsp baking soda

- ¾ cup egg whites

- ½ tsp vanilla extract

Procedure:

1. Place the pan over medium heat.

2. Mix all of the dry ingredients in a bowl.

3. Whisk the wet ingredients together in a bowl.

4. Gently add the wet and dry ingredients together.

5. Add enough coconut oil in a pan.

6. Pour the batter and spread it out into a pancake shape.

7. Cook for 4 minutes on the first side and flip. Cook for another 2 minutes.

8. Repeat the process until the batter is used up.

Chapter 3: Cookies

Double Chocolate Cherry Cookies

Ingredients:

- 1 ½ cups blanched almond flour

- ½ tsp baking soda

- ½ cup grape seed oil

- 1 tbsp vanilla extract

- 1 cup dried fruit juice sweetened cherries

- ½ tsp sea salt

- ¼ cup unsweetened cocoa powder

- ¾ cup agave nectar

- 1 cup coarsely chopped dark chocolate

Procedure:

1. Preheat the oven.

2. Place parchment papers on the baking sheets.

3. Mix the almond flour, cocoa powder, salt and baking soda in a large bowl.

4. Combine the grape seed oil, vanilla extract and agave nectar in a separate bowl.

5. Combine the wet mixture to the almond flour mixture.

6. Add the cherries and chocolate.

7. Spoon one tablespoon of dough into the baking sheet.

8. Space each cookie about 2 inches from each other.

9. Bake for 15 minutes until the top of the cookies are dry but not overly cooked.

10. Allow the cookies to cool on the rack for 20 minutes before serving.

Snicker Doodles

Ingredients:

- 2 cups fine ground almond flour

- ¼ tsp baking soda

- ¼ cup mild honey

- 1/3 cup melted palm shortening

- 1 ½ tbsp vanilla extract

For the cinnamon coating:

- 2 tbsp ground cinnamon

- 2 tbsp raw coconut crystals

Procedure:

1. Preheat the oven to 350 degrees.

2. Place parchment paper on the baking sheet.

3. Combine and stir the dry ingredients together in a medium bowl.

4. In a separate bowl, combine the vanilla, oil and honey.

5. Add the wet ingredients to the flour mixture and stir to combine. Allow to rest for few minutes until it thickens.

21

6. Combine the sugar crystals and ground cinnamon in a bowl.

7. Use clean hands or a rounded spoon to scoop dough. Gently form it into a ball and roll it in your palms. Sprinkle with the cinnamon mixture.

8. Place the balls into the baking sheet lined with parchment paper.

9. Space each ball about 3 inches apart.

10. Flatten the cookie with your hand.

11. Bake in the oven for 8 minutes at 350 degrees.

12. Leave the cookies on the baking sheet and allow to cool.

Walnut Cherry Almond Flour Cookies

Ingredients:

- 3 cups almond flour

- ½ cup butter

- 1/3 cup applesauce

- ½ tsp baking powder

- 2/3 cup dried cherries

- 1/3 cup dark chocolate chips

- ½ cup sugar

- ½ tsp salt

- 1 tsp vanilla

- 2/3 cup chopped walnuts

Procedure:

1. Preheat the oven to 350 degrees.

2. Mix the almond flour, applesauce, butter, salt, vanilla, baking powder and sugar in a food processor and blend until it is smooth.

3. Add the cherries, chocolate chips and walnuts.

4. Scoop the dough into your palm and form into balls.

5. Bake the balls for 15 minutes. Remember to watch it closely because it tends to brown quickly.

6. Place on the rack to cool.

Chocolate Dipped Walnut and Currant Cookies

Ingredients:

- 3 cups chopped walnuts

- ½ cup almond flour

- 1/3 tsp pure stevia extract

- 1/8 tsp sea salt

- 2 whisked eggs

- 1 cup pecans

- 6 tbsp coconut palm sugar

- ¼ tsp ground cinnamin'1/2 cup currants

- 1 tsp pure vanilla extract

For Dipping

- ½ tsp coconut oil

- 4 oz dark or semisweet chocolate

Procedure:

1. Preheat the oven to 350 degrees.

2. Line the baking sheet with parchment paper then set aside.

3. Process the walnuts and pecans until it has the same texture as a meal. Continue to pulse until the mixture clumps together.

4. Add the nut mixture to a medium bowl and combine with the almond flour, cinnamon, salt and sweetener. Mix to combine.

5. Stir in the currants, vanilla and egg until you have dough.

6. Scoop the batter and shape into balls. Flatten the dough ball slightly.

7. Bake for 15 minutes until the edges are golden and slightly firm.

8. Remove from the oven and place on a rack to cool.

9. Heat the coconut oil and chocolate in a broiler until it is fully melted. Dip one side of the cookies in the chocolate and place on the parchment paper.

10. Sprinkle with powdered sugar if desired.

11. Place in the refrigerator to harden.

Gingerbread People

Ingredients:

- 8 tbsp butter or coconut oil

- 1/3 cup honey

- ½ tsp allspice

- ½ tsp ground cloves

- 1/8 tsp sea salt

- 1 egg

- 3 cups almond flour

- 1 tsp ground ginger

- ½ tsp cinnamon

- 1 tsp baking soda

Procedure:

1. Combine the salt, flour, spice and baking soda together in a bowl.

2. Add the rest of the ingredients. Stir it until the dough is formed.

3. Form one large dough or two medium sized balls.

4. Freeze in the refrigerator for 30 minutes.

5. Preheat the oven at 350 degrees.

6. Place parchment paper above and below the dough to prevent it from sticking.

7. Spread some almond flour below the dough.

8. Roll and shape the cookies.

9. Gently place the cookies on the baking sheet.

10. Bake for 10 minutes until the edges are brown.

11. Place in a warm oven for 20 minutes.

12. Allow to cool before decorating.

Toffee Almond Flour Cookies

Ingredients:

- ½ cup softened butter

- 1 egg

- ½ tsp salt

- 3 cups almond flour

- ½ cup sugar

- 1 tsp vanilla extract

- ½ tsp baking soda

- ¾ cup toffee bits

Procedure:

1. Preheat the oven to 375 degrees.

2. Cream the sugar and butter for 3 minutes.

3. Add the egg and vanilla. Beat the mixture until the ingredients are well incorporated. Add this to the almond mixture.

4. Add the baking soda and salt and stir together. Add to the almond mixture.

5. Gently add toffee bits.

6. Scoop about one and one half tablespoon of the mixture into the baking sheet. You can also use an ice cream scooper to transfer the mixture to the baking sheet.

7. Smooth out the dough to make the cookies.

8. Bake for 10 minutes at 375 degrees.

9. Allow to cool for 5 minutes before serving.

Peanut Butter Almond Flour Cookies

Ingredients:

- ½ cup almond flour

- ½ tsp baking soda

- 1 egg

- 1 tsp vanilla extract

- ¼ cup sugar

- ½ tsp salt

- 1/3 cup peanut butter

Procedure:

1. Preheat the oven.

2. Combine the sugar, baking soda, salt and almond flour.

3. Beat the egg, peanut butter and vanilla.

4. Gently add the wet ingredients to the mix using your hands.

5. Divide the mixture in half and repeat the process until you have 8 sections.

6. Roll each section into dough. Use a fork to push the cookie down and make a cross pattern.

7. Bake the cookies for 11 minutes.

8. Place on the cooling tray for half an hour before serving.

Chapter 4: Main Dish

Shrimp Cake

Ingredients:

- 1 lb peeled and deveined shrimp

- 1 minced garlic clove

- 1 tbsp lime juice, freshly squeezed

- ½ tsp Celtic sea salt

- 1 egg

- ½ cup blanched almond flour

- 1 red or yellow bell pepper, chopped

- 2 tbsp thinly sliced scallions

- 1 tbsp agave nectar

- ¼ tsp chipotle chili, ground

- ½ cup finely chopped cilantro

- 3 tbsp grape seed oil

Procedure:

1. Place the shrimp in a blender then process until it is finely chopped.

2. Mix the shrimp, scallions, agave, lime, garlic, bell pepper, salt, egg, chipotle and cilantro in a large bowl.

3. Form the mixture in thick patties and coat with the almond flour.

4. Pour one tablespoon of the oil in a large pan.

5. Add the patties to the pan and cook for about 5 minutes per side until it is brown.

6. Remove and place on top of paper towels.

7. Repeat the procedure with the rest of the cakes.

Cod Piccata

Ingredients:

- 1 ½ lb cod

- ½ tsp Celtic sea salt

- 5 tbsp grape seed oil or butter

- ¼ cup lemon juice

- ¼ cup fresh chopped parsley

- ½ cup blanched almond flour

- ½ tsp all-purpose chef's shake

- 5 tbsp all olive oil

- 1 cup chicken stock

- ¼ cup brined capers

Procedure:

1. Chop the cod into 6 pieces.

2. Combine the salt, chef's shake and flour in a bowl.

3. Rinse the fish in cold water then dip into the flour mixture. Roll to coat.

4. Heat the oil in a pan over medium heat. Add half of the fish pieces and cook well for 3 minutes per side.

5. Transfer the fish to a plate. Cook the rest of the cod.

6. Place the plate of cod in the oven then start to prepare the sauce.

7. Add the lemon juice, stock and capers into the pan. Scrape the brown bits at the bottom to incorporate it to the sauce.

8. Reduce the sauce by half then add the remaining grape seed oil.

9. Place in a plate then pour the sauce over then sprinkle with parsley.

10. Serve warm.

Chicken Parmesan

Ingredients:

- 4 boneless and skinless chicken breast

- 2 eggs, whisked

- 7 oz tomato paste

- 1 tsp herbes de provence

- 16 oz mozzarella cheese

- 2 cups blanched almond flour

- 6 tbsp salted butter

- 2 cups water

- 6 sliced garlic cloves

Procedure:

1. Slice the chicken in half to have thinner cutlets. Pat it dry then set aside.

2. Dip the chicken in egg and allow the excess to drain. Coat it with the almond flour.

3. Melt the butter in a pan then cook the chicken until it is golden brown on both sides.

4. Place the chicken on a paper towel to drain.

5. Combine the tomato paste, herbs, water and garlic in a pan. Allow to simmer for 15 minutes.

6. Place half cup of tomato sauce in a baking dish.

7. Spread the chicken in a single layer then pour the tomato sauce and top with the mozzarella.

8. Bake for 10 minutes at 400 degrees.

9. Serve warm.

Salmon Wasabi Burgers

Ingredients:

- 1 lb skinless salmon fillet

- ¼ tbsp fresh ginger, peeled and minced

- ¼ cup fresh cilantro

- 1 tbsp freshly squeezed lime juice

- 1 tsp Celtic sea salt

- 1 tbsp water

- 1 tbsp fresh ginger

- ¼ cup freshly minced cilantro

- ½ cup blanched almond flour

- ¼ cup wasabi powder

- Coconut oil for frying

Procedure:

1. Rinse the salmon and pat it dry with paper towels.

2. Slice the salmon into ¼ inch cubes.

3. Mix the ginger, cilantro, lime juice, egg, salt, scallion and salmon in a large bowl.

4. Mix the wasabi powder and water in a small bowl to make a paste.

5. Pour the paste into the salmon mixture.

6. Shape the batter using your hands.

7. Pour the oil in a pan then place over medium heat.

8. Cook the patties until golden brown.

Fish Sticks

Ingredients:

- 1 lb white fish

- 1 cup blanched almond flour

- 6 tbsp olive oil

- 2 whisked eggs

- 1 tsp Celtic sea salt

-

Procedure:

1. Rinse the fish in cold water and place in a plate.

2. Chop the fish into 5 pieces. Make sure to follow the lines of the dish and remove any bone in the process. Place the eggs in a dish and mix with the flour and salt.

3. Heat the oil in a pan. Place over medium heat.

4. Place the fish sticks in the pan. Make sure to space them properly.

5. Cook for few minutes on each side until brown.

6. Add the oil to the pan and cook the remaining sticks.

7. Serve with tomato sauce or ketchup.

Chicken Piccata

- 4 boneless skinless chicken breast halves

- ½ tsp Celtic sea salt

- 5 tbsp grape seed oil

- ¼ cup lemon juice

- ¼ cup brined capers

- ½ cup blanched almond flour

- ½ tsp chef shake

- 5 tbsp olive oil

- 1 cup chicken stock

- ¼ cup fresh chopped parsley

Procedure:

1. Slice the chicken horizontally and cut them in butterfly. Cut them in four pieces if the chicken is too large.

2. Place the chicken in a parchment paper and use a skillet to pound it until it is about ¼ inch thick.

3. Combine the chef's shake, flour and salt in a bowl.

4. Wash the chicken in water and dip in the flour mixture until it is well coated.

5. Heat the oil in a large pan and place it in medium heat. Add half of the chicken. Cook each side for about 3 minutes.

6. Transfer the chicken to a plate then continue to cook the remaining pieces.

7. Place the chicken in a warm oven.

8. Combine the chicken stock, capers and lemon juice in a pan. Use a spatula to loosen the bits and incorporate it to the sauce.

9. Whisk the sauce until it is reduced by half.

10. Transfer to a plate then pour the sauce over it.

11. Garnish with parsley before serving.

Chicken Meatballs

- 1 cup chopped zucchini

- ½ cup coarsely chopped parsley

- ¼ cup blanched almond flour

- 1 lb boneless skinless chicken breast

- ½ tsp ground pepper

- 1 cup chopped carrots

- 3 medium garlic cloves

- 1 egg

- 1 tsp Celtic sea salt

Procedure:

1. Preheat the oven to 350 degrees.

2. Combine the carrots, garlic, zucchini and garlic in a food processor then blend well together.

3. Add the egg, flour and chicken to the mixture. Pulse it to combine.

4. Season it with salt, pepper and chili powder. Process until well combined.

5. Scoop a tablespoon sized mixture and shape it into meatballs. Place on top of the baking sheet.

6. Bake the meatballs for 25 minutes until firm and brown.

7. Serve with your favorite sauce.

Chapter 5: Cakes

Flourless Lemon Almond Cake

Ingredients:

- 4 eggs, yolks and whites separated

- ¼ tsp ground cardamom

- 1 ½ cup finely ground almond flour

- 1 tsp cider vinegar

- 1 tsp baking powder

- 2 tbsp lemon zest, packed

- ½ cup white sugar

- Pinch of salt

- Powdered sugar for sprinkling

Procedure:

1. Preheat the oven to 350 degrees and line the pan with parchment paper. Grease the sides with butter.

2. Beat the egg yolk, half the sugar (1/4 cup) and lemon zest in a large bowl.

47

3. Stir together the cardamom, baking powder and almond flour in a separate bowl. Add to the egg yolk mixture. Beat until combined.

4. Beat the egg whites in a clean bowl with an electric mixture. Tip: try using a cold glass or metal bowl. Start the speed low and gradually increase. When you notice bubbles forming in the mixture, add the salt and vinegar. Once the whites increase in volume, gradually add the remaining sugar (1/4 cup). Beat the egg white mixture until soft peaks form.

5. Gently pour the egg white mixture into the almond mixture a little bit at a time. Fold together the ingredients.

6. Carefully spoon the mixture into prepared pan.

7. Bake it for 35 minutes or until it is firm to the touch. Allow to cool slightly and remove from pan.

8. Serve at room temperature with powdered sugar sprinkled over the top.

Source: simplyrecipes.com

Simple Summer Peach Cake

Ingredients:

- 3 ripe peaches

- 1 cup sugar

- 1 large egg

- ½ tsp vanilla extract

- ½ cup almond flour

- ¼ tsp baking soda

- ¾ tsp finely ground nutmeg

- 6 tbsp softened unsalted butter

- ½ cup buttermilk

- ¼ tsp almond extract

- 1 cup all-purpose flour

- 1 tsp baking powder

- Turbinado sugar

Procedure:

1. Preheat the oven and grease the cake pan with butter.

2. Slice the peaches into small bite size pieces. Toss the peaches with the sugar and nutmeg. Set this aside.

3. Cream the butter and sugar using a wooden spoon. Add the extract, egg and buttermilk. Stir to mix.

4. Mix the baking powder, salt, flours and baking soda. Add the flour mixture to the butter and stir until smooth. Pour this mixture into your prepared pan.

5. Press the peaches into the cake. You can arrange them into a certain patter or you can simply scatter them on top. Sprinkle the sugar on top.

6. Bake the cake for 10 minutes. Reduce the heat to 325 degrees and bake for another 45 minutes. Bake until done.

Blackberry and Almond Coffee Cake

- 1 ½ cups all-purpose flour

- 1 tsp baking powder

- ¼ tsp salt

- 1 cup granulated sugar

- 1 cup sour cream

- ½ cup almond flour

- ½ tsp baking soda

- ½ cup unsalted butter, softened

- 2 eggs

- 1 tsp vanilla extract

For the Filling:

- 1 ½ cup blackberries

- ¼ cup sugar

- ¼ cup water

- 2 tbsp cornstarch

For the Topping:

- ½ cup flour

- 3 tbsp granulated sugar

- 1 cup slivered almonds, chopped

- 1/3 cup brown sugar

- 4 tbsp melted unsalted butter

Procedure:

1. Make the filling by mixing the water, cornstarch and sugar in a pan. Cook and stir for 5 minutes or until the mixture is thick and bubbly.

2. Place the almonds, sugar, and sugar in a bowl and whisk to combine properly. Drizzle the butter on top and toss to combine until large chunks are formed. Set this aside.

3. Preheat the oven to 350 degrees. Grease the pan with cooking spray and dust it with flour.

4. Sift the baking soda, salt, flour and baking powder.

5. Use a beater to cream the sugar and butter. Add the eggs one at a time. Mix until it is well incorporated before adding the next egg.

6. Add the sour cream and mix. Add the flour and mix again. Avoid over mixing since this can make your batter lumpy.

7. Pour half of the mixture into the pan and spread it using a spatula. Pour the blackberry filling on top and sprinkle the streusel.

8. Bake for 40 minutes at 350 degrees until it is done. Cake is ready when it is free of crumbs.

Zucchini Almond Cake

Ingredients:

- ½ stick unsalted butter, melted plus 5 tbsp, room temperature

- ¼ tsp fine salt

- ½ cup packed light brown sugar

- 1 cup finely grated zucchini, squeezed of excess liquid

- 1/3 cup confectioner's sugar

- ¼ cup plus tbsp potato starch

- 3 large eggs, room temperature

- 4 tsp pure vanilla extract

- 1 ½ cups almond flour

- 8 oz cream cheese, room temperature

Procedure:

1. Preheat the oven and grease the pan with butter. Line it with parchment paper or butter paper.

2. Combine the potato starch, salt, baking powder and almond flour in a bowl.

3. Place a heatproof bowl with an inch of simmering water. Add the eggs and whisk it until foamy.

4. Add the sugar and continue to whisk until the sugar is completely dissolved and the mixture is fluffy. Whisk on high heat until it is thick and pale.

5. Use a rubber spatula to beat the butter, vanilla and cream cheese together until it is fluffy. This will take about 3 minutes.

6. Add the confectioner's sugar and beat to combine. Spread on top of the cake.

Chocolate Buckwheat Cake

Ingredients:

- 6 oz bittersweet or semi-sweet chocolate

- 4 large eggs, separated

- 1/3 cup plain whole milk yogurt

- ½ tsp salt

- ¼ cup buckwheat flour

- ½ cup unsalted butter, cubed

- ½ cup unrefined sugar

- 1 tsp vanilla extract

- ¾ cup almond flour

Procedure:

1. Preheat the oven. Spread butter into the cake pan and line it with parchment paper.

2. Set a large ovenproof bowl over simmering water. Melt the chocolate and butter until it is smooth. Remove from the heat and allow to cool slightly.

3. Mix the egg yolks, sugar, vanilla, salt and yogurt in a bowl. Add the melted chocolate. Stir in the almond flour and buckwheat flour.

4. Whip the egg whites until soft peaks are formed. Fold one third of the egg whites into the chocolate mixture to lighten it before adding the remaining chocolate mixture. Stir well until combined.

5. Scrape the batter into the pan and bake for another 25 minutes until the cake is set. The cake should still be soft. Allow to cool for 10 minutes before removing from the cake pan.

Christmas Cake

Ingredients:

- 1 large orange
- ¾ cup agave nectar or honey
- 2 cup blanched almond flour
- 1 tsp baking soda
- ½ cup dried apricots, chopped
- ½ cup walnut, chopped
- 4 eggs
- ½ tsp almond extract
- ½ tsp Celtic sea salt
- 1 cup dried cranberries
- ½ cup chopped pistachios

Procedure:

1. Wash the orange and boil it in a pan whole until it is soft.
2. Place the orange in a food processor and blend it until smooth.

3. Process the almond flour, agave, eggs, almond extract, salt and baking soda until it is well blended.

4. Transfer to a mixing bowl and add the apricots, pistachios, cranberries and walnuts.

5. Pour the mixture in a pan that is greased with butter and dusted with almond flour.

6. Cover with tin foil once the cake is brown on top.

7. Bake for 45 minutes at 350 degrees until done.

8. Allow to cool for 2 hours before serving.

Cherry Blueberry Crumble

Ingredients:

- 4 cups fresh cherries, pitted

- ¼ cup agave nectar or honey

- 1 tbsp vanilla extract

- 1 pint fresh blueberries

- 1 tbsp lemon juice

- 2 tbsp arrowroot powder

For the Topping:

- 2 ¼ cups blanched almond flour

- 1/3 cup grape seed oil

- ¼ tsp Celtic sea salt

- ¼ cup agave nectar or honey

Procedure:

1. Place the cherries and blueberries in a dish.

2. Sprinkle the lemon juice, vanilla, agave then stir with the arrowroot.

3. Make the crumble in a large bowl and combine the almond flour and salt.

4. In a small bowl, mix the grape seed oil and agave.

5. Mix the wet and dry ingredients together to form the topping.

6. Crumble the topping over the fruit mixture.

7. Cover and bake it for an hour at 350 degrees until bubbling.

8. Uncover and bake for few minutes until the top is golden brown.

9. Remove from the oven before serving.

Conclusion

Thank you again for purchasing *"**Almond Flour Recipes for Optimal Health and Quick Weight Loss**: Gluten Free Recipes for Celiac Disease, Gluten Sensitivities, and Paleo Free Diets!"*

I hope this book was able to help you to make delicious dishes with almond flour. What I hope even more for you is that you lose the weight you desire!

Losing weight and changing your lifestyle isn't easy. We all need motivation to keep our goal in mind.

Finally, if you enjoyed this book, please take the time to share your thoughts and post a review on Amazon. It'd be greatly appreciated!

I would love for you to share your experiences, stories and encouragements with me. My email address is emmarosekindle@gmail.com

In addition, please remember to check out our Facebook page in order to find other resources and upcoming promotions:

https://www.facebook.com/joypublishing

With sincere thanks,

Emma Rose

Preview Of "Paleo Free Diet Guide for Beginners: Over 50 Paleo Free Diet Recipes for Fast Weight Loss and Optimal Health"

Introduction

I want to thank you and congratulate you for purchasing the book, *"Paleo Free Diet Guide for Beginners: Over 50 Paleo Free Diet Recipes for Optimal Health and Fast Weight Loss"*.

This book contains everything you might need to know when it comes to getting started with the Paleo diet. It is provided in an easily digestible format that allows you to better absorb the information. There are no complicated explanations about how it works! You'll be given what you need straight up so you won't have to waste time trying to understand exactly what the diet is. Whether it's for your overall good health or to lose a few pounds, Paleo can certainly help you with it. To help you get started, we'll do the same and start you off with 50 of the best Paleo recipes that you can slowly but surely shift your everyday menu to.

It's never easy changing a diet. I often fall into self pity when I can no longer have the foods I enjoy. Either I feel sorry for myself or I get rebellious and binge and anything and everything. I always knew the value of eating healthy. I could just never bring myself to do it. It wasn't until I had a miscarriage that I got serious about my health. I have made drastic changes that others just don't understand. But the pay off is the weight I've lost and the better health I'm experiencing.

My hope for you is not to be on another "diet." This isn't a restriction diet like Atkins. The goal is to have a lifestyle change. Lifestyle changes are more sustainable and maintain weight loss long term compared to restriction diets. The change is hard to start but worth it when you commit. The trick is to get the momentum to start.

Thanks again for purchasing this book. I hope you enjoy reading it and eating the recipes from it!

With gratitude,

Emma Rose

Chapter 1 – What Is the Paleo Diet?

The Paleo Diet is known by many names such as the cavemen diet, stone age diet and hunter-gatherer diet, to name a few. The concept behind this diet follows that of the Paleolithic era before the development of agriculture. Essentially, you consume the same foods that the cavemen used to eat. The focus is on eating food closest to its natural, unprocessed state. The cavemen would gather their food from any source available whether it was wild animals, berries, vegetables, or fruits. As a result, they were strong, fit, and healthy for thousands of years.

This type of diet is still very young, less than fifty years only, but more in depth researches and studies are being conducted to increase the information and knowledge on this diet. The results of previous studies conducted on the Paleo diet reveal the improvement of health to the people involved. This is attributed to the fact that no processed foods and additives are included. The Paleo Diet is a diet that works with our genetics – before machinery and processing got involved. Foods that were not available during the Paleolithic time such as dairy products, salt, sugar and grains are not included in the preparation of the Paleo diet.

The modern diet predominately consumed in the Western world is full of refined foods, trans fats, salt and sugar. These ingredients are known to indirectly cause diseases such as hypertension, diabetes, strokes, obesity and other heart problems. The list goes on even further with the increase diagnosis of cancer, Parkinson's, Alzheimer's, depression and infertility. "What an extraordinary achievement for a civilization: to have developed the one diet that reliably makes its people sick!" (Michael Pollen, Food Rules: An Eater's Manual, Penguin Books 2009).

Foods included in the Paleo Diet

- Fruit

- Vegetables

- Lean Meat

- Seafood

- Nuts/Seeds

- Healthy Fats (eg. coconut, avocado, nuts and seeds, olive oil, grass fed butter)

Foods NOT included in the Paleo Diet

- Dairy

- Grain

- Processed Food

Check out the rest of "Paleo Free Diet Guide for Beginners: Over 50 Paleo Free Diet Recipes for Fast Weight Loss and Optimal Health" on Amazon.

Or go to:http://amzn.to/1jIJUFX

Coconut Flour Recipes for Optimal Health and Quick Weight Loss

Gluten Free Recipes for Celiac Disease, Gluten Sensitivities, and Paleo Free Diets

Emma Rose

Table of Contents

Introduction

I want to thank you and congratulate you for purchasing the book, **"Coconut Flour Recipes for Optimal Health and Quick Weight Loss**: *Gluten Free Recipes for Celiac Disease, Gluten Sensitivities, and Paleo Free Diets"*.

This book contains proven steps and strategies on how to integrate coconut flour into your diet for a healthier food lifestyle.

In this book, you will learn about the benefits of using coconut flour and how it can help you lose weight and become healthier without limiting the food you're eating. I have also included several guilt-free coconut flour recipes that you and your loved ones will surely enjoy.

Thanks again for purchasing this book, I hope you enjoy it! Please take some time to stop by and LIKE our Facebook page:

https://www.facebook.com/joypublishing

With gratitude,

Emma Rose

Chapter 1: Why Use Coconut Flour?

Nowadays, people are getting more conscious about their food lifestyle and how it affects their overall well-being. Most of the foods that are available today are processed or refined however there are some good alternatives that can be used without taking away much from flavor.

Among the healthy alternatives for refined grains is the coconut flour. Coconut flour is one of the best alternatives to replace the usual refined wheat flour. Since coconut flour is very versatile, it can be used to replace refined grains from almost all kinds of baked goods and meals.

There are five major advantages in using coconut flour:

1. Coconut flour is gluten free. For people who have allergies or are sensitive to gluten, coconut flour is definitely a gift from heaven. By using coconut flour, people allergic to gluten will be able to enjoy baked treats.

2. Coconut flour improves cell regeneration. This type of flour has high non-gluten protein content that helps improve the growth of cells and rejuvenation.

3. Coconut flour is high in fiber. For people who want to lose or maintain their weight, coconut flour is a good alternative ingredient to make your own breads and cakes without feeling guilty about it. Foods made with coconut flour makes a person feel fuller faster and longer.

4. Coconut flour has high manganese content which means this ingredient will enable you to absorb more nutrients from foods faster. Also, manganese

is proven to promote healthy blood sugar levels and thyroid health.

5. Coconut flour contains lauric acid. This healthy saturated fat is important to a person's immune health and it promotes healthy skin.

Though coconut flour can be used as a substitute ingredient to almost all recipes calling for wheat flour, it also takes some tweaking with the other ingredients for it to work well with baking and cooking. For example, coconut flour is drier than wheat flour therefore it requires more water when used in baking. The following are recipes that you can use to start your journey to a healthier you.

Chapter 2: Coconut Flour Bread Recipes

Zucchini Bread

Ingredients:

- ½ cup of coconut flour

- ¾ tsp of baking soda

- ½ tsp of salt

- 1 tbsp of cinnamon

- ½ tsp of nutmeg

- 4 pcs of pasture-raised eggs

- 3 tbsp of raw honey OR grade B maple syrup

- 1 cup of zucchini, shred it finely

- 1 pc of ripe banana, mashed

- 1 tbsp of coconut oil

- ½ cup of walnuts

Procedure:

1. Turn on the oven and set it to 350F.

2. Prepare a loaf pan and grease it with coconut oil. You can also line the pan with parchment paper, if available. Set the pan aside.

3. Prepare a piece of cheesecloth or a nut milk bag and place the finely shredded zucchini inside. Squeeze as hard as you can to remove the excess moisture from the zucchini.

4. In a large mixing bowl, combine the egg, honey or maple syrup, and banana. Mix together until the ingredients are well-incorporated.

5. Add in the coconut flour, baking soda, salt, cinnamon, and nutmeg into the mixing bowl and mix well. Then, add in the shredded zucchini and stir until the mixture becomes smooth.

6. Add in the walnuts and stir.

7. Pour the batter into the loaf pan and place it inside the oven. Bake for 45 to 50 minutes or until the bread has completely set.

Coco Doughnuts

Ingredients:

- ½ cup of coconut flour

- ¼ tsp of sea salt

- ¼ tsp of baking soda

- 6 pcs of eggs

- ½ cup of honey

- 1 tbsp of vanilla

- ½ cup of unsalted butter OR coconut oil, already melted

- 5 tbsp of honey

- Coconut flakes for toppings

Procedure:

1. Turn on the oven and set it to 350F.

2. In a mixing bowl, combine the coconut flour, sea salt, and baking soda. Stir the dry ingredients together until well-mixed.

3. Add in the eggs, honey, vanilla, and butter into the mixing bowl. Use a whisk or a hand mixer set on low to blend all of the ingredients together.

4. Prepare about 8 donut pan circles and fill each pan with the batter about 2/3 of the way.

5. Place the donut pan circles into the oven and bake for 20 minutes.

6. While baking, warm 5 tablespoons of honey and place it in a saucer. Then, toast the coconut flakes.

7. Dip each piece of donut in the honey and sprinkle it with the toasted coconut flakes.

Coco Bread

Ingredients:

- ¾ cup of coconut flour

- 1 tsp of baking soda

- A pinch of sea salt

- 4 pcs of whole eggs

- 3 pcs of eggs, white and yolk separated

- 5 tbsp of organic butter

- 3 tbsp of coconut milk

- 1 tbsp of raw honey

- Organic virgin coconut oil

Procedure:

1. Prepare a loaf pan and lightly grease it using the coconut oil. Then, line the loaf pan with baking paper with a coating of coconut oil just to make sure that the loaf does not stick to the pan.

2. Turn on the oven and set it to 350F.

3. Take the egg whites from three eggs and whisk it until it become stiff. You can use a hand mixer if you like. Set it aside.

4. Take the egg yolks and pour it in a food processor. Add in the four whole eggs, organic butter, coconut milk, and raw honey. Blend the ingredients until thoroughly combined.

5. Add in the coconut flour, baking soda, and salt gradually into the food processor while blending. Continue to process the ingredients until the mixture becomes thick in consistency.

6. Prepare a large mixing bowl and pour in the mixture from the food processor. Take the egg whites and fold it in the mixture.

7. Once the mixture and egg whites are thoroughly combined, pour in the batter into the loaf pan. Place the pan inside the oven and bake for 40 minutes.

8. Reduce the heat to 300F and cover the loaf pan. Cook for another 5 to 10 minutes.

9. Once cooked, remove the loaf pan from the oven and place it on a cooling rack to cool completely before slicing and serving.

Chocolate Muffin

Ingredients:

- ½ cup of coconut flour

- 1 tsp of baking soda

- A dash of salt

- ¼ cup of coconut sugar

- 2 tbsp of cocoa powder

- 1 tsp of vanilla extract

- ¼ cup of coconut oil

- 2/3 cup of coconut milk

- 4 pcs of pastured eggs

- 1 tsp of apple cider vinegar

Procedure:

1. Turn on the oven and set it to 350F.

2. Melt the coconut oil and place it in a bowl or a food processor. Add in the coconut flour, baking soda, salt, coconut sugar, cocoa powder, vanilla extract, coconut milk, eggs, and apple cider vinegar. Stir or blend the ingredients together until it forms a smooth batter.

3. Prepare a muffin tin and line it with paper or silicone liners.

4. Pour the batter about ¾ of the way of each muffin liner as the muffin will rise once it is cooked.

5. Place the muffin tin inside the oven and bake for 20 to 30 minutes.

Cheese Biscuits

Ingredients:

- 1/3 cup of coconut flour

- ¼ cup of butter, melted

- 4 pcs of eggs

- ¼ tsp of salt

- ¼ tsp of cream of tartar

- 1/8 tsp of baking soda

- ½ cup of shredded cheddar cheese

- ¼ cup of shredded parmesan cheese

Procedure:

1. Turn on the oven and set it to 400F.

2. In a mixing bowl, combine the coconut flour, salt, cream of tartar, and baking soda. Stir and make a well in the center of the dry ingredients.

3. Add in the eggs and melted butter in the center of the dry ingredients and mix. Whisk the ingredients together until it forms a smooth batter.

4. Add in the cheeses and stir to properly combine.

5. Prepare a baking sheet and spray it with cooking spray. Drop spoonfuls of batter into the sheet at even intervals.

6. Place the baking sheet inside the oven and bake for 8 to 10 minutes. Once cooked, let it cool on a wire rack then remove the biscuits from the baking sheet.

Gingerbread Doughnuts

Ingredients:

- 4 pcs of large eggs

- ¼ cup of melted coconut oil

- 1/3 cup of coconut palm sugar

- ¼ cup of full fat coconut milk

- 2 tbsp of blackstrap molasses (unsulphured)

- 1 tsp of raw apple cider vinegar

- 1 ½ tsp of pure vanilla extract

- 1 ¾ tsp of ground cinnamon

- 1 ¼ tsp of ground ginger

- 1 tsp of ground cloves

- ¾ tsp of allspice

- ½ tsp of baking soda

- ¼ tsp of freshly ground nutmeg

- ¼ tsp of sea salt

- 1/8 tsp of cayenne pepper

- ½ cup of coconut flour, sifted

- ½ cup of organic powdered sugar

- 2 tbsp of full fat canned coconut milk

- ¼ tsp of pure vanilla extract

- A pinch of sea salt

Procedure:

1. In a mixing bowl, combine the eggs, melted coconut oil, and palm sugar. Use a hand mixer to beat the ingredients together.

2. In a small bowl, combine the coconut milk, apple cider vinegar, molasses, and vanilla extract. Stir the ingredients together until properly combined. Pour the mixture into the large mixing bowl and beat until the ingredients are well mixed.

3. In a separate small bowl, combine the ground ginger, ground cloves, ground cinnamon, allspice, nutmeg, baking soda, cayenne pepper, and sea salt. Stir the ingredients together. Add in the spice mixture into the mixing bowl and stir until all the ingredients are just combined.

4. Add in the sifted coconut flour into the mixing bowl and use the hand mixer to incorporate all the ingredients. Blend until it forms a smooth batter.

5. Turn on the oven and set it to 350F.

6. Pour the batter into a doughnut pan and place it inside the oven. Bake for 18 to 20 minutes then place it immediately on a cooling rack.

7. While waiting for the doughnuts to cool, prepare a large mixing bowl and combine the organic powdered sugar, coconut milk, vanilla, and salt. Whisk the ingredients together until no lumps are present.

8. Use a spoon to drizzle the glaze over the doughnuts.

Lemon Bread with Lemon Glaze

Ingredients:

- 6 pcs of eggs

- ¼ cup of coconut oil, melted

- Zest of 2 pcs of lemons

- Juice from 2 lemons combined with coconut milk to make 1 cup

- 1/3 cup of honey

- 2/3 cup of coconut flour

- 1 tsp of baking soda

- ¼ tsp of salt

- 2 tbsp of coconut oil

- 2 tbsp of honey

- 2 tbsp of coconut milk

- Zest and juice of 1 lemon

- ½ tsp of vanilla extract

Procedure:

1. Turn on the oven and set it to 350F.

2. In a large mixing bowl, add in the eggs, ¼ cup of coconut oil, zest from 2 pieces of lemons, 1 cup of the lemon juice and coconut milk mixture, 1/3 up of honey, coconut flour, baking soda, and salt. Whisk the ingredients together until it forms a smooth batter.

3. Prepare a loaf pan and grease it with coconut oil. Pour the batter into the pan and place it inside the oven. Bake for 32 to 45 minutes then remove from the oven and set it aside to cool completely.

4. In a small bowl, combine the 2 tablespoons of coconut oil, 2 tablespoons of honey, 2 tbsp of coconut milk, zest and juice of 1 lemon, and vanilla extract. Whisk together until well-incorporated then pour the glaze on top of the loaf.

5. Place the loaf inside the refrigerator for about 30 minutes to help the glaze set before serving.

Chapter 3: Coconut Flour Breakfast Recipes

Coconut Porridge

Ingredients:

- ½ cup of full-fat canned coconut milk

- ¼ cup of water

- 3 tbsp of coconut flour

- 2 tbsp of finely shredded coconut

- ½ of a banana, mashed

- Frozen berries or chopped nuts, will be used for toppings

Procedure:

1. Prepare a small saucepan and add in the coconut milk, water, coconut flour, and the finely shredded coconut. Stir the mixture and let it boil.

2. Place a lid and reduce the heat. Let it simmer for 2 to 3 minutes stirring occasionally.

3. Remove the saucepan from the heat and add in the mashed banana. Whisk to combine and stir.

4. Replace the saucepan into the stove and cook for another 2 minutes. Continue stirring until it thickens.

Coconut Bake

Ingredients:

- 6 tbsp of coconut flour

- 10 pcs of eggs

- 2 tsp of vanilla extract

- 4 pcs of ripe bananas, mashed

- ¼ tsp of salt

Procedure:

1. In a mixing bowl, add in the coconut flour, eggs, vanilla extract, mashed bananas, and salt. Mix the ingredients thoroughly and let it sit for 10 minutes.

2. Prepare a muffin tin by lining it with muffin liners. Then, pour the batter into the tin.

3. Place the muffin tin inside the oven and bake for 20 to 25 minutes at 350F. You can also bake this in your microwave for 3 minutes on high settings. Just remember to use ramekins instead of muffin tins.

Bacon Pancakes

Ingredients:

- 16 pcs of cooked bacon strips

- ¼ cup of mashed ripe banana

- 4 pcs of large eggs

- 6 tbsp of full fat canned coconut milk

- 1 tsp of apple cider vinegar

- 1 tsp of vanilla extract

- 3 tbsp of organic coconut flour

- 1 tsp of cinnamon

- ½ tsp of baking soda

- A pinch of salt

- Coconut oil

- 2 tbsp of maple syrup

Procedure:

1. Place the bacon on a wire rack and bake it in the oven for 10 to 20 minutes at 400F.

2. In a medium mixing bowl, combine the mashed banana, eggs, apple cider vinegar, coconut milk, and

vanilla. Whisk the ingredients together until properly combined.

3. In a separate mixing bowl, combine the organic coconut flour, baking soda, cinnamon, and salt. Give it a stir until the ingredients are incorporated.

4. Pour in the banana mixture into the coconut flour mixture and whisk together until the batter has no lumps.

5. Prepare a skillet and heat the coconut oil. Once the oil is hot, add in three tablespoons of batter into the pan. Make a rectangular shaped pancake about the size of your bacon. Flip the pancake once bubbles form on top.

6. Repeat the process until all the batter is cooked then assemble the pancakes. Place strips of bacon on top of a pancake then drizzle with a bit of maple syrup. Put another pancake on top and enjoy.

Strawberry Flapjacks

Ingredients:

- 1 pc of egg

- 1 tbsp of almond flour

- 1 tsp of coconut flour

- Coconut oil

- ¼ tsp of baking soda

- ½ tsp of cream of tartar

- Stevia

- Organic strawberries

Procedure:

1. Prepare a skillet and heat the coconut oil.

2. In a small bowl, whisk the egg and adding in a splash of water. Once combined, add in the almond flour and coconut flour and whisk again.

3. Add in the baking soda, stevia, and cream of tartar. Mix the ingredients together until it forms a smooth batter. You can taste the batter to gauge the amount of stevia needed.

4. Slice the strawberries into thin slices.

5. Pour the batter into the pan to make one mini-pancake. Once the pancake is slightly firm, place strawberry slices on top. Flip the pancake to cook the other side.

Oats and Flax Crisps

Ingredients:

- 2/3 cup of rolled oats

- 1/3 cup of flax seeds

- ½ cup of shredded coconut

- ¼ cup of coconut oil, melted

- 1/3 cup of unsweetened coconut milk

- 3 tbsp of maple syrup

- 2 tbsp of coconut flour

- 1 tbsp of coconut sugar

- 1 tbsp of chia seeds

- 3 tsp of ground ginger

- 1 tsp of cinnamon

- 1 tsp of pure vanilla extract

- ¼ tsp of salt

Procedure:

1. Turn on the oven and set it to 350F. Prepare two baking sheets and line it with silicone mats or parchment paper.

2. In a large mixing bowl, combine the rolled oats, flax seeds, shredded coconut, coconut flour, coconut sugar, chia seeds, ground ginger, cinnamon, and salt. Stir the ingredients together until evenly combined.

3. In a separate bowl, combine the coconut oil, coconut milk, maple syrup, and vanilla extract. Stir the ingredients until well-mixed. Then, pour the mixture over the dry ingredients. Stir the ingredients together until properly incorporated.

4. Drop a spoonful of the mixture into the baking sheets and flatten it with the back of the spoon to make thin biscuit-like crisps.

5. Place the baking sheets in the oven and bake for 18 to 25 minutes. Once cooked, remove the baking sheets from the oven and set it aside to cool completely.

Chapter 4: Coconut Flour Cake Recipes

Apple and Cinnamon Cake

Ingredients:

- 6 pcs of free-range eggs

- 1 cup of coconut oil OR organic butter, already melted

- ¼ cup of raw honey

- 1 pc of apple, grated

- Zest of 1 pc of lemon

- ½ cup of coconut flour

- 1 cup of desiccated coconut

- 2 tsp of cinnamon

- 1 tsp of baking soda

- A pinch of sea salt

- 1 pc of apple, slice it into very thin wedges

- Juice of ½ of a lemon

- Extra coconut flour for dusting

Procedure:

31

1. Turn on the oven and set it to 150C.

2. Prepare a cake tin and spray it with cooking oil. You can also line it with parchment paper if you prefer.

3. In a food processor, add in the eggs, coconut oil, honey, grated apple, lemon zest, coconut flour, desiccated coconut, cinnamon, baking soda, and sea salt. Blend all of the ingredients together until properly combined.

4. Spoon the batter into the cake tin and spread it evenly.

5. Arrange the wedges of apples on top of the batter. Decorate it however you like. Then, squeeze the lemon juice on the apples.

6. Place the cake tin inside the oven and bake for 45 minutes.

7. Once cooked, let it cool complete before transferring it into a serving plate. Dust with the extra coconut flour before serving.

Coffee Cake

Ingredients:

- 1 cup of coconut flour
- ½ tsp of Celtic sea salt
- 1 tsp of ground cinnamon
- 8 pcs of large organic eggs
- 1 tsp of baking soda
- ½ cup of strained plain coconut milk yogurt
- 5 tbsp of coconut oil
- ½ cup of honey
- 1 tbsp of vanilla extract
- 1 ½ cups of nuts
- 2 tsp of cinnamon
- 4 tbsp of honey
- 4 tbsp of cold coconut oil, cut it into tablespoons

Procedure:

1. Turn on the oven and set it to 325F. Place the rack in the middle part of the oven.

2. In a food processor, combine the coconut flour, sea salt, 1 teaspoon of ground cinnamon, eggs, baking soda, coconut milk yogurt, 5 tablespoons of coconut oil, ½ cup of honey, and vanilla extract. Blend the ingredients until the mixture becomes smooth.

3. Prepare an 8" x 8" baking dish and pour in the batter inside.

4. Wash and dry the food processor bowl. Add in your choice of nuts, 2 teaspoons of cinnamon, 4 tablespoons of honey, and 4 tablespoons of coconut oil. Process until the nuts are coarsely chopped and all of the ingredients bind together.

5. Spoon the topping on the batter and spread it across the surface of the batter.

6. Place the baking dish in the oven and bake for 40 to 45 minutes. Once cooked, place it on a wire rack and let it cool for about 20 minutes before cutting and serving.

Chocolate Cake

Ingredients:

- ¾ cup of coconut flour, sifted
- ¼ cup of cacao powder
- 1 tsp of Celtic sea salt
- 1 tsp of baking soda
- 10 pcs of eggs
- 1 cup of coconut oil
- 1 ½ cups of coconut sugar
- 1 tbsp of vanilla extract
- ¼ tsp of orange zest
- 1 cup of dark chocolate
- ½ cup of grapeseed oil
- 2 tbsp of agave nectar
- 1 tbsp of vanilla extract
- A pinch of Celtic sea salt

Procedure:

1. In a small mixing bowl, combine the coconut flour, cacao powder, Celtic sea salt, and baking soda. Mix the ingredients together.

2. In a large mixing bowl, combine the eggs, coconut oil, coconut sugar, vanilla extract, and orange zest. Use a hand mixer to mix the ingredients until properly incorporated.

3. Gradually add in the dry ingredients mixture into the large bowl while blending with the hand mixer.

4. Prepare two 9" round cake pans. Lightly grease it with oil and dust using the coconut flour. Pour the batter inside the cake pans and place it inside the oven.

5. Set the oven to 325F and bake for 35 to 40 minutes.

6. Once cooked, remove from the oven and place it on a cooling rack to cool completely.

7. Prepare a small saucepan and add in the dark chocolate and grapeseed oil. Combine the two ingredients over low heat.

8. Add in the agave nectar, vanilla extract, and salt into the saucepan. Stir until the ingredients are well-incorporated.

9. Remove from the heat and place it inside the freezer for about 15 minutes.

10. Once cool, remove the frosting from the freezer and use the hand mixer to whip the frosting until it becomes thick and fluffy.

11. Place the frosting in between the two layers of cakes. Place one cake on top of the other and use the remaining frosting to cover the top of the cake.

Double Chocolate Beet Root Brownies

Ingredients:

- 4 pcs of large pastured eggs

- 1/3 cup of coconut oil, melted

- 1 tsp of vanilla extract

- ¾ cup of maple syrup

- 1 ½ cups of beet puree

- 2 tbsp of coconut cream

- ½ cup of coconut flour

- ½ cup of raw cocoa powder

- ½ tsp of unrefined salt

- ½ tsp of baking soda

- ½ cup of chocolate chips

Procedure:

1. Turn on the oven and set it to 350F.

2. In a large mixing bowl, combine the eggs, coconut oil, vanilla extract, maple syrup, beet puree, and coconut cream. Use a hand mixer to thoroughly mix the ingredients.

3. In another bowl, combine the coconut flour, cocoa powder, salt, baking soda, and chocolate chips. Stir to mix the ingredients together.

4. Gradually add in the dry ingredients into the large mixing bowl containing the wet ingredients. Use the hand mixer to properly combine the ingredients.

5. Prepare an 8" x 8" baking pan and grease it lightly with coconut oil. Then, pour the batter into the pan.

6. Place the baking pan inside the oven and bake for 35 to 40 minutes.

Pumpkin Bars

Ingredients:

- 1 ½ cups of pumpkin puree

- ¾ cup of coconut flour

- ¾ cup of maple syrup

- 1 ½ tsp of ground cinnamon

- ¾ tsp of ground ginger

- ¼ tsp of ground cloves

- ¾ tsp of baking soda

- ¼ tsp of salt

- 2 pcs of large eggs

- Coconut oil

Procedure:

1. Turn on the oven and set it to 350F.

2. Prepare a 9" x 9" baking dish and lightly grease it using the coconut oil.

3. In a large mixing bowl, combine the pumpkin puree, coconut flour, maple syrup, ground cinnamon, ground cloves, ground ginger, baking soda, salt, and eggs. Stir the ingredients together until well-incorporated.

4. Pour the batter into the baking dish and smooth the top. Place the baking dish inside the oven and bake for 40 to 45 minutes. Once cooked, let it cool completely before cutting and serving.

Chocolate Chip Banana Cookies

Ingredients:

- 1 pc of ripe banana

- 1 pc of large egg

- 2 tbsp of extra virgin coconut oil

- 3 tbsp of coconut flour, sifted

- 1 tbsp of vanilla extract

- ½ tsp of cream of tartar

- 1/8 tsp of baking soda

- 1/8 tsp of sea salt

- ¼ cup of chocolate chips

Procedure:

1. Turn on the oven and set it to 325F.

2. Prepare a baking pan and line it with parchment paper.

3. In a large mixing bowl, combine the banana and egg. Use a hand mixer to mix the ingredients together. Slowly add in the coconut oil while mixing.

4. Add in the coconut flour, vanilla extract, cream of tartar, baking soda, and sea salt. Blend the ingredients until it forms a smooth batter.

5. Add in the chocolate chips into the batter and stir.

6. Use a spoon to drop about 1 inch balls of batter on the baking pan then flatten the batter to form a cookie shape. Leave enough space between each cookie.

7. Place the baking pan inside the oven and bake for 40 minutes.

Classic Vanilla Cake

Ingredients:

- 4 pcs of large eggs, whites and yolks separated

- 1 tsp of cream of tartar

- ¼ cup of extra virgin coconut oil

- 3 tbsp of raw honey

- ¼ cup of coconut flour, sifted

- 2 tsp of vanilla extract

- ¼ tsp of baking soda

- 1/8 tsp of salt

Procedure:

1. Turn on the oven and set it to 350F.

2. Prepare an 8" x 1.5" round cake pan and line it with parchment paper.

3. In a large mixing bowl, combine the cream of tartar with the egg whites. Use a whisk or a hand mixer to whip the ingredients together to form stiff peaks.

4. In a separate mixing bowl, combine the honey and coconut oil. Use a hand mixer to mix the two ingredients to form a cream. Add in the egg yolks, and mix again.

5. Gradually add in the coconut flour, vanilla extract, baking soda, and salt into the mixture. Use the hand mixer to combine the ingredients until it forms a smooth batter.

6. Pour the batter into the bowl with the whipped egg whites and fold until properly incorporated. Pour the mixture into the cake pan.

7. Place the cake pan in the oven and bake for 20 minutes.

Lady Finger Cookies

Ingredients:

- 4 pcs of pastured eggs, separate the white from the yolk

- ¼ cup of maple syrup

- ¼ tsp of baking soda

- ½ tsp of vanilla extract

- 1/3 cup of coconut flour, sifted

- 1 tsp of freshly ground coffee

Procedure:

1. Turn on the oven and set it to 400F.

2. Place the egg whites in a mixing bowl and beat it until stiff peaks form using a hand mixer.

3. In a large mixing bowl, add in the egg yolks, vanilla extract, baking soda, and maple syrup. Whisk the ingredients together until properly combined. Add in the sifted coconut flour and continue to mix the ingredients until it forms a smooth batter.

4. Fold the egg whites into the mixture then add in the ground coffee.

5. Prepare a baking sheet and line it with parchment paper. Pour the batter into a pipe bag and attach a round pipe tube at the end. Make about 3-in long cookies on the baking sheet.

6. Place the baking sheet inside the oven and bake for 13 minutes. Once down, set it aside to cool completely before serving.

Custard Cake

Ingredients:

- 4 pcs of eggs

- 2 cups of milk

- ½ cup of coconut flour

- ½ cup of raw honey

- 1 tsp of pure vanilla extract

- 2 tsp of baking powder

- ¼ cup of butter, melted

- 1 ½ cups of unsweetened coconut flakes

- ½ cup of chocolate chips

Procedure:

1. Turn on the oven and set it to 350F.

2. In a large bowl, add in the eggs, coconut flour, milk, honey, vanilla extract, baking powder, and butter. Whisk the ingredients together until it forms a smooth batter. You can use a hand mixer if you prefer.

3. Add in the chocolate chips and coconut flakes. Stir until all ingredients are properly combined.

4. Prepare an 8" cake pan and pour the batter inside. Place the pan inside the oven and bake for 45 to 50 minutes.

5. Once cooked, let it rest and cool completely before splicing and serving.

Conclusion

Thank you again for purchasing "**Coconut Flour Recipes for Optimal Health and Quick Weight Loss**: *Gluten Free Recipes for Celiac Disease, Gluten Sensitivities, and Paleo Free Diets*"!

I hope this book was able to help you to discover the benefits of using coconut flour.

The next step is to enjoy the recipes you have learned to make healthier foods for yourself and your loved ones.

Losing weight and changing your lifestyle isn't easy. We all need motivation to keep our goal in mind.

Finally, if you enjoyed this book, please take the time to share your thoughts and post a review on Amazon. It'd be greatly appreciated!

I would love for you to share your experiences, stories and encouragements with me. My email address is emmarosekindle@gmail.com

With sincere thanks,

Emma Rose

Preview of "Clean Eating Guide: Lose Weight Quickly, Achieve Optimal Health and Feel Energized with Clean Eating for Busy Families and Clean Eating Recipes

Chapter 1

What Is Clean Eating?

You have probably come across the term 'clean eating' but you are still not familiar about its exact meaning. This is being used by people who work in the health and fitness industry such as personal trainers ad dietitians. People who are health conscious and workout fanatic also often use this word. Does it have something to do with cleaning the food before eating or cooking? Or maybe it has something to do with the kind of food that you eat.

The loose definition of clean eating is eating food in its most natural state. These days, people are starting to pay more attention to the kinds of food that they eat and how these foods are made. They take note of the food's ingredients and make sure that the food product only contains all natural ingredients.

The term clean eating first came out in the 1990s. Today, it is still being used by health conscious individuals from different backgrounds and culture to refer to the kind of all natural diet that they have. The definition of clean eating can vary from person to person. Some define clean eating as eating mostly fruits and vegetables while others define it as not eating anything artificial. You will find out more about these things as you read this book.

What Clean Eating is not?

If you think clean eating is another diet program, like the South Beach diet or Paleo diet, you are wrong because clean eating is a way of life. It also does not follow any strict rules about what food group to eat and not to eat, how many calories you should consume in a meal, and so on. This is the most basic way of healthy eating that promotes weight loss and boost energy. Everybody can do this, even those who are not trying to lose weight.

Clean eating will not make you feel deprived or frustrated because it is so easy to follow. You do not even need to have a really strong determination because it is all a matter of choosing natural over artificial.

Is there such a thing as 'dirty' eating?

You are probably wondering if there is such a thing as 'dirty' eating or the opposite of clean eating. Clean eating does not literally mean eating foods that have less dirt. It means that you are choosing the best and healthiest food choices from different food groups in their most natural state. 'Dirty' eating is not the opposite of clean eating because there is no such thing as eating dirty. The opposite of clean eating is choosing the wrong food to eat and eating junk foods and processed foods that leave toxins in your body.

Clean eating also looks at the source of food. It should not come from large commercial manufacturers that use machines to process food. The foods that clean eaters usually use come from small farms that do not use chemicals and undergo processes. This is why clean eating is often associated with organic eating.

Check out the rest of "Clean Eating Guide: Lose Weight Quickly, Achieve Optimal Health and Feel Energized with Clean Eating for Busy Families and Clean Eating Recipes" on Amazon

Or go to: http://amzn.to/UVzNER

Check Out My Other Books

Below you'll find some of my other books also available on Amazon and Kindle. Search for these titles on the Amazon website to find them.

Paleo Free Diet Guide for Beginners: Over 50 Paleo Free Recipes for Optimal Health & Fast Weight Loss

Paleo Desserts: Satisfy Your Sweet Tooth With Over 100 Quick & Easy Paleo Dessert Recipes & Paleo Baking Recipes

Raw Food Diet Guide: Lose Weight Quickly, Achieve Optimal Health & Feel Energized with the Raw Food Diet & Raw Food Recipes

Clean Eating Guide: Lose Weight Quickly, Achieve Optimal Health & Feel Energized with Clean Eating For Busy Families & Clean Eating Recipes

Alkaline Diet Guide: Lose Weight Quickly, Achieve Optimal Health & Feel Energized with the Alkaline Diet & Alkaline Recipes

Coconut Flour Recipes for Optimal Health & Quick Weight Loss: Gluten Free Recipes for Celiac Disease, Gluten Sensitivities & Paleo Free Diets

Almond Flour Recipes for Optimal Health & Quick Weight Loss: Gluten Free Recipes for Celiac Disease, Gluten Sensitivities & Paleo Free Diets

Wheat Free Diet for Beginners: Lose Weight Quickly, Achieve Optimal Health & Feel Energized with Gluten Free Recipes for Celiac Disease, Gluten Sensitivities & Paleo Free Diets

Detox Diet Guide: Lose Weight Quickly, Achieve Optimal Health & Feel Energized Through the 10 Day Detox

Sugar Detox Guide for Beginners: Lose Weight Quickly, Achieve Optimal Health, Feel Energized & Eliminate Sugar Cravings Naturally

Ketogenic Diet Guide for Beginners: How to Achieve Rapid Weight Loss, Optimal Health & Unstoppable Energy with Ketogenic Diet Recipes

Anti Inflammatory Diet for Beginners: Lose Weight Fast, Optimize Health, Slow Aging, Fight Inflammation, Conquer Pain & Increase Energy with the Anti Inflammation Diet Recipes

One Last Thing...

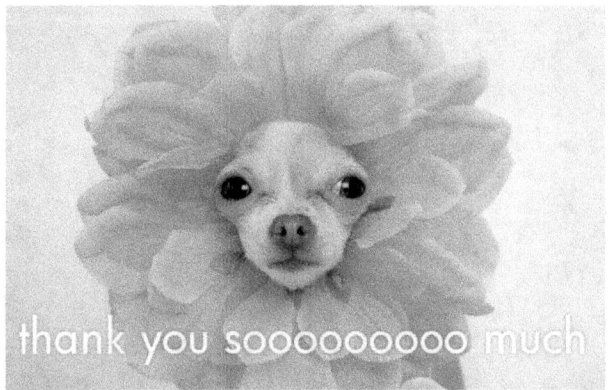

If you believe that this book is worth sharing, would you please take the time to let others know how it affected your life? If it turns out to make a difference in the lives of others, they will be forever grateful to you, as will I.

www.ingramcontent.com/pod-product-compliance
Lightning Source LLC
Chambersburg PA
CBHW060358290526
45791CB00002B/556